I0765811

LOQUAIMAT DIET

Eat your way to weight loss

Takehiro Mia

Foreword

When you think about following a diet, you may think of depriving you of your favorite foods, Have you ever imagined that you eat all kinds of food and do not follow the strict rules of dieting, yet you lose weight and improve your health?

I was reading about the diet of luqamiat in the past few months and I was really excited to experienced it.

However, I could not find any sources concerning the diet plan or how the diet work out. So that, I have decided to take the challenge and do lot of researchers in order to clarify the notion of luqaimat's diet to many people who are interested in losing weight.

The main reason that drove me to write this book is to share my experience and show the world that this diet helped me to lose weight successfully. I would like to mention that weight loss is not my only reason that pushes me to share my own experience, but writing this book has been basically to let people know the advantages of this diet which I am going to state later on.

Table of content

Introduction

There are two top ranking diet plans that are based on portion control, namely: Jenny Craig and SlimFast.

Jenny Craig: combines personalized counseling (over the phone and in person) with prepackaged portion-controlled meals.

SlimFast: is portion control diet depending on branded snacks and shakes. The modified SlimFast advise the dieters to eat six times a day - three snacks, two SlimFast shakes or bars and one 500-calorie meal. The expected weight loss is about 10% of body weight loss in six months.

Luqaimat diet is the portion control diet of the Arab world. It has four major advantages over the abovementioned highly ranked and famous Jenny Craig and SlimFast diets.

1. Luqaimat diet creates results outperform all other comprehensively well-known diets. For the patient with BMI around 40, weight reduction after 1.5 years adds up to 30.5% of the patients' average original weight. These outcomes surpass

by a wide margin the consequences of 8% and 10% created from Jenny Craig and SlimFast, individually.

2. Luqaimat diet does not require specific meals or prepackaged foods. The dieter can eat any food he wishes as long as it is in small portions.

3. Luqaimat diet raises the self-esteem and confidence because the dieter will be trained on delayed gratification, which in turn will potentiate his decision making abilities.

4. Luqaimat diet can be maintained for long since all kinds of food are allowed. Hundreds of my patients are still following Luqaimat diet since 2005.

Luqaimat is an Arabic word for the minimum amount of food in one´s diet that must be eaten in order to keep fit. I innovated my Luqaimat diet in 2005, the diet plan advise the dieters to eat 5 Luqaimat each day in addition to one moderate-size diversified meal.

Each Luqaimat may be a single piece of fruit, vegetable, a small piece of bakery, sweets, or chocolate, or five units of nuts, and so on, repeated every 2 – 4 hours. The moderate-size diversified meal consists of 3 plates the first contains a maximum of 1.5 cup-full of starchy food and vegetables plus palm-sized meat, poultry or fish. The second plate contains a maximum of 1.5 cup-full of green salad, and the third plate contains a matchbox size of sweets.

In my opinion, Luqaimat diet plan is the perfect formula for weight loss due to many reasons including the following:

1. Obese people are allowed to eat all their favorite foods (but in small volumes), so they can maintain their diet for good and stick to it.
2. Obese patients are educated about the action of Luqaimat on their gut and brain, so they will reach better mind-gut cooperation.
3. Obese people are trained on satiating gradually their stomach through boosting frequently Elhashemy´s Stomach Satiety Spot "ESSS", so within few weeks, they will not need to eat big volumes of food.

4. Obese people are trained on regenerating gradually their brown fat through eating frequently purple fruits and vegetables laden with anthocyanins (according to Elhashemy´s theory of brown adipose tissue regeneration).

All these reasons result in unprecedented success rate in weight loss using Luqaimat diet plan. This is why, tens of thousands of obese and super obese patients in Egypt and the Arab world are following my diet plan instead of going on globally famous diets, or being submitted to bariatric surgery.

The study of the Dr. Elhashemy

Dr. Elhashemy started his underlying examination with 313 of his patients. Throughout year and a half, he tested them to eat as few luqaimats as could be allowed, however the same number of as they required, alongside moderate meals containing two measures of green salad of mixed greens with one tablespoon of olive oil, 1/2 measures of vegetables and starch, one bit of meat and a little treat. Dr. Elhashemy arranges a luqaimat as a little organic product or vegetable serving, three to five nuts, a small baked good or a bit of chocolate.

a. **Benefits:**

Dr. Elhashemy reports that by eating luqaimats, his patients did not require substantial meals for the duration of the day, and therefore, they shed 70 to 103 percent of their excess weight. Every patient lost a normal of four kilograms every month and along these lines kept up a BMI of 25 amid the year and a half in which the investigation was directed.

b. **Considerations:**

As Dr. Elhashemy explains, psychology plays an important role in a successful Luqaimat Diet. Patients must understand that although they may still crave food, luqaimats should provide the energy they need while suppressing the hunger hormone, ghrelin. Overall, the diet is designed to train and acclimatize your brain to eating smaller portions by targeting its pleasure center with minimal doses of your favorite foods.

c. **Expert Insight:**

The Luqaimat Diet may also help people battle the need to eat more food in social situations. As Dr. Elhasmey explains, "I believe that seeing people eating large volumes of food encourages other people to imitate them, and these behaviors could lead them to enter a vicious circle. I believe that we can reverse this vicious circle by the Luqaimat Diet."

What is the luqaimat diet?

Luqaimat is a Mediterranean dessert, but it also has another meaning in Arabic, small piece of food.

Here I will explain the luqaimat Diet in detail.

Dr El hashemy is a physician professor at Cairo's University .And the diet centers on how decreasing the size of stomach by making it comfortable with small amounts of.

This diet does not take Calories into consideration; however the main pint to success in this diet is the amount of food eaten throughout the day.

The idea is very simple, and its success rate is very high to me and a lot of people here in Egypt (As Dr El Hashemy is Egyptian so was introduced in Egypt in 2005)

 Note: you may eat and follow everything listed her unless you have any health restrictions around it.

This is a diet to be accommodated to become a life style, you don't have to follow everything to the letter. You should always do what is best for your body and what you feel comfortable in.

All the world will be fat ... except people eating luqaimat

The conclusion of this analysis comes in line with several previous studies that warn of the repercussions of this worldwide obesity epidemic within the close to future.

The conclusion of this analysis comes in line with many previous studies that warn of the repercussions of this worldwide fleshiness epidemic at intervals the about to future.

Based on the expertise of Dr ELHASHEMY, he founds that reducing meal volumes is that the major think about managing obesity, which reducing meal volumes for long is best achieved by a semi-permanent coaching on small-volume meals ("Luqaimat"), until it becomes a habit.

Similar to drug addiction, uptake massive volumes of food stimulates the feeding centers of the brain resulting in longing for any larger volumes of food. He thinks that we are able to reverse this vicious circle by semi-permanent coaching on the small-volume meals (Luqaimat).

Luqaimat is an Arabic word for the minimum quantity of food that ought to be eaten so as to supply the specified energy. Every Luqaimat perhaps one fruit or vegetable, alittle piece of any store, sweets, or chocolate, or 3 to 5 units of nuts, and so on. Within the diet plan, he recommends to this patient to eat Luqaimat each 2- three hours.

This Luqaimat diet arrange permits for a moderate-sized meal, that consists of two cups of green salad with one table spoon of oil and dressing, 1.5 cups of vegetables and carbohydrates, one slice of animal protein (preferably fish or poultry), and one little piece of sweets.

In 2005, he started advising few many their patients to follow this Luqaimat diet plan.

In 2008, he postulated ther his theory of the presence of a satiety area at the gastric fundus that he named: Elhashemy's stomach satiety Spot "ESSS". This area is sensitive – according to his theory – to the bit applied to that by any solid food (such as almonds). this may stimulate the hypothalamic satiety center. after all the pathway is mediated through the vagus nerve fibers. This leads to early satiety, less intake of food, and consequently an excellent loss of weight.

In 2009, few thousands of obese Egyptians followed the Luqaimat diet plan with spectacular results that inspired additional individuals to follow this diet.

In 2010, many thousands of obese people in several Arab countries followed his innovated Luqaimat diet plan with nice success in losing their additional weight.

I hope that within the close to future Luqaimat diet, that proven to all or any whom have followed it to be the foremost convenient and healthiest diet plan, can facilitate in fighting the world's obesity epidemic.

Characteristics of the Luqaimat diet

The luqaimat diet characterized by many important features mentioned in the following points:

- A preferred diet for all those who want to lose excess weight as quickly as they are, because it is not a harsh diet or any fatigue or excessive effort.

- One of the most effective and safest forms of dieting on all body organs.

- It is one of the most successful dieting systems due to its guaranteed results and the loss of lost weight.

- The Luqaimat system treats many colon problems such as bloating and gas.

- Eliminate feelings of deprivation and hunger, where individuals eat all meals, but in small amounts.

- weight loss did not stop but lasted for many months until most of the class has succeeded in reaching the ideal weight, and even that many obese overweight people lose more than 132 pounds a year after the application of this diet

- Pregnant women can follow the diet without any harm to their health and the health of the fetus, taking into account the intake of vitamins containing the necessary nutrients for the fetus such as milk, fish and the multiplication of fruits.

- Also, there are no contraindications to follow this diet in the case of breastfeeding, so it is necessary to increase the intake of large amounts of water (8 cups) daily.

- The person who obeys the system of Luqaimat shows that it is a lifestyle rather than a normal diet

How to apply the Luqaimat diet!

This diet will consist of a happy meal (as lunch or dinner) and 5 luqaimat (Pieces of food), between each luqaima and the other you'll have 2-3 hours and this should be organized.

If you eat before the 2 hours have past then you may disrupt the system and if you stay longer than 3 hours then your body may enter starvation mode and store anything you eat afterwards as fats.

The diet of Luqaimat consists of three basic parts:

1. Small frequent meals (Five or more a day)

- Fruits

- A vegetable of any kind
- A cup of popcorn
- A small piece of Dark Chocolate
- A cup of yogurt
- 5 biscuits
- Half a cup of soup
- Half cup of ice cream
- Half a can of tuna (Take out the extra oil)
- ¼ a sandwich from any fast food restaurant
- Half a large fish
- Half a cup of cornflakes
- 1/3 of a hand piece of cake
- 5 of any nuts
- Half a cup of milk
- Half a bag of chips
- Cup of salad
- Boiled egg
- Fat - free chicken steak
- A cup of sugar.
- A cup of fresh juice

- A cup of Nescafé (this considered a luqaima when there's milk and sugar is it's black then it's not considered as a Luqaima)

- Half a slice of pizza.

- 0.5 Cup of milk.

- 3 Balms or dates.

- Half a mango fruit equals half a cup.

- 2 Figs.

- 2 apricot.

- Cup of pomegranate.

- Strawberry Cup.

- A cup of cherries.

- A cup of pineapple.

- A glass of watermelon.

- Cup of cantaloupe.

- A banana.

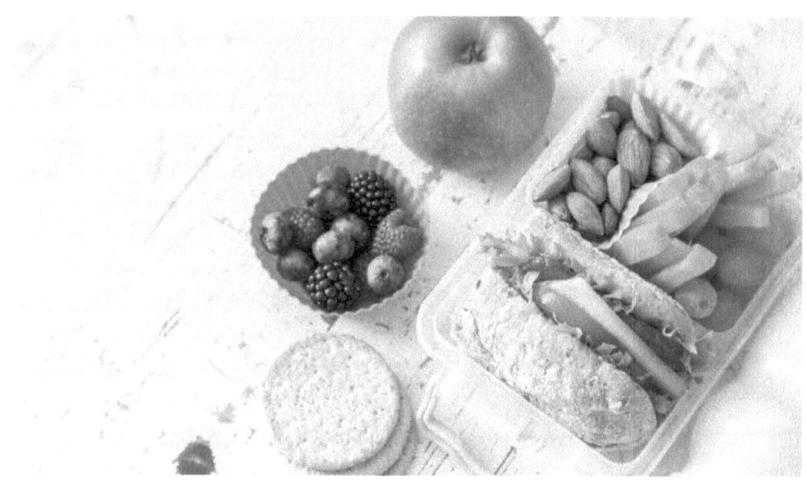

In general you can eat the amount of cup of any food you want, taking into account eating greasy food once a day no more and taking two to three times the fruit of the same kind.

These are examples but you should follow through any other type of food.

These are considered as the snacks to be eaten throughout the day.

2. HAPPY MEAL

This basically consists of:

A cup and half: salad and any liquids (soup and drink) distribute as you wish but must have a portion of salad.

A cup and half of hot food: this can be divided as a cup of carbohydrates, half a cup of cooked vegetables, slice (half a cup) of protein.

A dessert the size of a small match box (eat this without feeling guilty at all!)

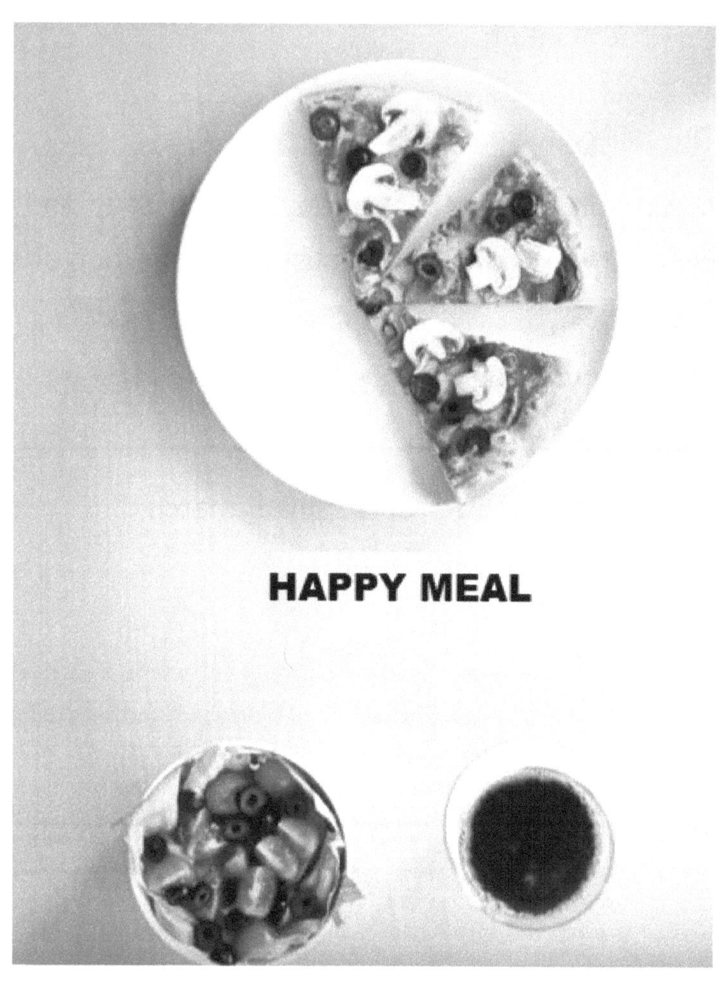

✓ This is for those who weighed less than 198lb

- ✓ If he weighed between 198lb and 330lb, I would advise him to take one and a half times the above.

- ✓ If he weighs more than 330lb, I advise him to take twice the amount of the meal for people under the weight of 198lb.

When the weight of the patient declines to a lower level, the amount of food in the main dish will also be reduced to the lowest level.

3. Almonds or peanuts

The goal of the third part of the diet is to increase the activity of the point of ELHashemy full stomach "ELHASHEMY STOMACH SATIETY SPOT", so I recommend that follow the diet of lactate eat a glass of water or any other drink first and then after 10 minutes, eating 3 almonds or 5 grains of peanuts and every hour for four to Five consecutive hours before the meal.

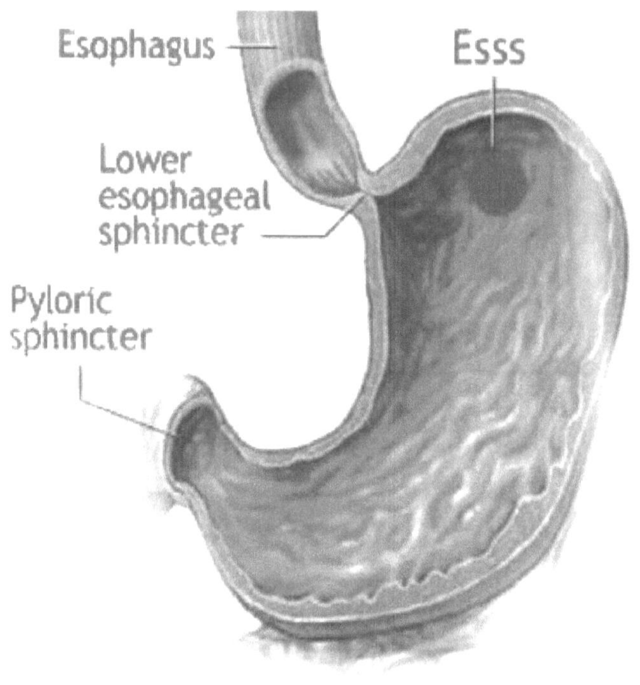

ELHASHEMY STOMACH SATIETY SPOT

What we change to come back to our graceful bodies again!!

Obesity has spread in the world like an epidemic, and I think the main reason is that people have changed their habits, they have acquired many bad habits, the most important of which is eating large amounts of food.

For our bodies to be graceful again, we have to change our life style.

1. Psychological preparation before sitting at the dining table, eat a meal with a maximum of three cups.

2. Do not eat or drink in front of television, so that we eliminate the link between eating and the

movement of the mouth while watching television.

3. We train every day for at least 5 Luqaimat and thus become psychologically accustomed to eating small portions of food.

4. To eat 5 peanuts or 3 almonds 7 consecutive times to activate ELHashemy stomach satiety spot that helps us feel full when eating the meal.

5. To move permanently at home and at work.

6. Take care to accompany those who struggle like us to get rid of excess weight.

7. To sleep at least seven hours, because there is a direct relationship between the decline in the number of hours of sleep and obesity.

- This is due to an increase in the hormone ghrelin.
- Decreased activity level due to fatigue.
- Decreased degree of mental concentration, this eliminates the ability of the mind to control the amounts of food eaten by humans.

Scientific objectives of the luqaimat

The diet luqaimat aims to:

1. To create a state of visual familiarity "visual cues" with the very small sizes of food so that these sizes are normal for man.
2. Create a state of psychological acceptance "psychological cues" for those small sizes of food.
3. A state of neurodevelopmental normalization of this method in the memory center of the brain "Hippocampal Neuroplasticity" so that the execution is done automatically.
4. A state of repeated stimulation of the skinny gene this gene was discovered by a scientist for nearly fifty years and then discovered by two scientists in

2007 is present in human cells. But none of the scientists succeeded in finding how to activate it, in the opinion of Dr. ELHASHEMY that eating these Luqaimat provokes the skinny gene more than full hunger.

5. The occurrence of repeated inhibition of the hormone Ghrelin produced by the lining of the stomach every three or four hours when there is no food, but if it reached the food, even a small amount, the stomach reduces secretion hormone.

    Ghrelin is a hormone that is produced and released mainly by the stomach with small amounts also released by the small intestine, pancreas and brain.

6. To create a state of psychological sense of food security, the realization that a person will eat a large number of Luqaimat, up to 70 small meals a week will remove the anxiety of the lack of the number of meals.

7. Adjust **the fat set point**[1] in the brain to the required weigh, because the use of frequent Luqaimat frequently leads to slowing the hunger hormone "Ghrelin" and at the same time to increase the satiety hormone and burn energy "leptin", reducing the point of weight in the brain to normal weight.

---

[1] https://curiosity.com/topics/your-weight-has-a-set-point-that-your-brain-thinks-is-best-curiosity/

Luqaimat and human memory

Whenever a person thinks about food, whether in terms of quantity or quality, or even if he remembers the smell or taste of food, he craves this food eager to get it in any way, and then he will ask large quantities to satisfy the various brain centers related to feeding, reward.

Fast-food chain owners have realized the important link between the large meal and the brain-reward center. These companies are tempting consumers to large volumes so that these volumes of memory are linked to the psychological satisfaction of the three brain centers associated with eating, so they lower the prices of these large meals to encourage demand.

As for those who are trained in luqaimat lifestyle, the memory of food will not affect him very much, because he will eat only a small part when he asks for this desired food.

Food and human genes

Before the beginning of the 21st century, scientists believed that genes within cells were fixed for life, so they believed there was no hope of changing them.

After the beginning of this century, it became clear that genes change according to the impact of the environment and the impact of different types of foods and the impact of human behavior.

The most obvious interpretation of this phenomenon is the entry of fast food in human alimentation in the present time, has changed his lifestyle and they tend to eat psychologically and crave to taste, but they have inherited their love for their children, and this is conclusive evidence that the repetition of food type and size leads to a state of habitual it ,Dr. ELhashemy noted that obese patients who were trained on Luqaimat in 2005 had turned their genes in they became in 2008 do not eat only small portion and do not care about the large food sizes that they ate previously.

Benefits of non-diversity in Luqaimat

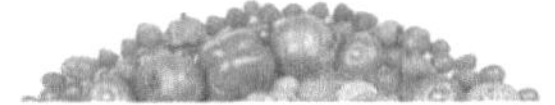

When we eat ten meals a day consisting of only two varieties, this does not require a larger amount of food.

A large number of Luqaimat a day gives a person a sense of food security, he usually does not ask for more.

 The small size of the veggies and their non-diversity makes the happy meal a feast for them, even if the size is small.

There is a lot of research for scientists that the lack of diversity of food leads to a reduction of interest in the request of large quantities of it.

The success of the Luqaimat system begins when the three methods converge

The science of Luqaimat contains three ways that converge together after three months of implementation.

The first: Luqaimat diet

Each day only two varieties, every category 4-5 times in succession between once and the other 1.5-3 hours, with an average meal equivalent to the size of 3 cups and are taken last day or evening every day.

One of the two types as a fruit is preferred to be repeated four times as an antioxidant.

Eat 5 peanuts or 3 almonds per hour, for seven consecutive times or less depending on the time available.

An obese patient needs psychosocial support, so that, the idea of the lactate system can be established in his mind, with the point of satiety being strongly stimulated.

This support lasts about three months to achieve the best results, and some cases may require a full year to achieve a continuous decrease in weight 2lb per week, 104lb per year (in 25 weeks).

Those who hasten to lose weight quickly in the beginning, it completely eliminates the idea of stimulating the point of satiety and the idea of continuous psychological therapy does not work weight loss only in an orderly manner, and in most cases, they restore the weight lost before the end of the year.

How to overcome difficulties

Getting rid of obesity is very difficult, and maintaining the ideal new weight is more difficult, global studies have shown that more than 95% of the people were followed the world-famous regimens they failed to maintain their new weight and returned excess weight within two years at most.

The person applying this diet, the weight loss continued with him gradually and slowly, however, he did not recover any of the lost weight.

How does he get it when he eats small quantities of food barely enough to give him energy for only two or three hours?

How can he regain it as he clings to this unique system that makes him eat whatever he loves?

Despite these features of the Luqaimat diets, the human when he begins to apply this diet face several difficulties, including:

1. It goes back to breakfast, lunch, and dinner.
2. It may be forgotten in the midst of the work eating Luqaimat every two hours, increasing the secretion of the hunger hormone.
3. That coworkers may eat fast foods in front of him, the cannot resist the temptation to participate with them.

Therefore, who wants to lose weight completely and retain his weight throughout his life he should be to resist these difficulties gradually and helps him as follows:

1. Read some chapters of the book before going to sleep every night until the information of this diet is printed in his subconscious mind.

2. Training to eat a few peanuts or almonds and repeated every hour for seven consecutive hours at most.

3. Request support from a parent or friend or a nutritionist

4. If you eat a large meal in one of the banquets is not the end of the world, enough to stick to the Luqaimat in the following meals and continue to succeed in losing excess weight.

How to eat after reaching the desired weight

We must ask ourselves the following question:

What happens to an obese patient who has had a gastric bypass surgery or a Gastric stapling surgery?

The answer is that they continue their normal lives and the amount of food continues a few, because if the belt was removed or expanded to open their appetite again for large amounts of food.

Hence, the diet of lactate will become an automatic natural habit engraved in the memory of the person continues without thinking about it, and is characterized by the stomach belt that there is no foreign body in the abdomen and without complications.

Fasting and Luqaimat

Fasting is that the ancient secret of health. It's ancient as a result of it's been practiced throughout all of human history. It's a secret because this powerful habit has been nearly forgotten.

But currently many of us are re-discovering this dietary intervention. It will carry large advantages if it's done right: weight loss, accrued energy, reversal of kind a pair of diabetes and plenty of alternative things. Plus, you'll save time and cash.

Food is definitely accessible, however you select to not eat it. This could be for any amount of your time, from a number of hours up to days or maybe weeks on finish. You will begin a quick at any time of your selecting, and you'll} finish a quick at will, too. You'll be able to begin or stop a quick for any reason or no reason in the slightest degree.

Fasting has no customary length, because it is simply the absence of feeding. Anytime that you simply don't seem to be feeding, you're fasting. As an example, you will quick between dinner and breakfast successive day, an amount of roughly 12-14 hours. In this sense, fasting ought to be thought of an area of lifestyle.

Consider the term "break fast". This refers to the meal that breaks your fast – that is completed daily. Instead of being some style of cruel and strange penalization, country language implicitly acknowledges that fasting ought to be performed daily, although just for a brief length.

Fasting isn't one thing queer and curious, however an area of everyday, traditional life. It's maybe the oldest and most powerful dietary intervention possible. However somehow we've forgotten its awe-inspiring power and unheeded its therapeutic potential.

Learning the way to fast properly give us the choice of exploitation it or not.

At it's terribly core, fasting merely permits the body to burn off excess body fat. It's necessary to appreciate that this is often traditional and humans have evolved to quick while not prejudicial health consequences. Body fat is simply food energy that has been keep away. If you don't eat, your body can merely "eat" its own fat for energy. Life is regarding balance. The great and therefore the unhealthy. The rule and therefore the principle.

An equivalent applies to feeding and fasting. Fasting, after all, is just the flip facet of feeding. If you're not feeding, you're fasting.

Here's however it works:

When we eat, a lot of food energy is eaten than will instantly be used. A number of this energy should be keep away for later use. Insulin is that the key hormone concerned within the storage of food energy.

Insulin rises once we eat, serving to store the surplus energy in 2 separate ways that. Sugars may be joined into long chains, known as polyose so keep within the liver.

There is, however, restricted storage space; and once that's reached, the liver starts to show the surplus aldohexose into fat. This method is termed De-Novo Lipogenesis (meaning virtually creating Fat from New).

Some of this fresh created fat is keep within the liver, however most of it's exported to different fat deposits within the body. Whereas this is often a lot of sophisticated method, there's no limit to the quantity of fat which will be created. So, 2 complementary food energy storage systems exist in our bodies.

One is

definitely accessible however with restricted cupboard space (glycogen), and therefore the different is tougher to access however has unlimited space for storing (body fat). The process goes in reverse once we don't eat (intermittent fasting). Insulin levels fall, communication the body to start out burning keep energy as no a lot of is coming back through food. Blood sugar falls, that the body should currently pull glucose out of storage to burn for energy.

Glycogen is that the most simply accessible energy supply.

It's counteracted into glucose molecules to produce energy for the opposite cells. This will give enough energy to power the body for 24-36 hours. After that, the body can begin breaking down fat for energy.

So, that the body solely very exists in 2 states – the fed (insulin high) state and therefore the fasted (insulin low) state. Either we tend to are storing food energy, or we tend to are burning it. It's one or the opposite.

If feeding and fasting are balanced,
then there's no internet weight gain.
If we tend to begin feeding the minute we tend to roll out of bed, and don't stop till we tend to attend sleep, we tend to pay most our time within the fed state. Over time, we'll gain weight. We've not allowed our body any time to burn food energy. To restore balance or to lose weight, we tend to merely have to be compelled to increase the

quantity of your time we tend to burn food energy. That's intermittent fasting. In essence, fasting permits the body to use its keep energy. After all, that's what it's there for.

The necessary factor to know is that there's nothing wrong therewith. That's however our bodies are designed.

That's what dogs, cat, lions and bears do. That's what humans do.
If you're perpetually feeding, as is commonly counseled, then your body can merely use the incoming food energy and ne'er burn the body fat. You'll solely store it. Your body can reserve it for a time once there's nothing to eat. You lack balance. You lack fasting.

How do I break a fast with Luqaimat?

We start our breakfast with two cups:

- Cup water

- A cup of juice or milk.

After ten minutes

Our happy meal

Then we eat as usual regular one and the other 1.5 to 2 hours.

We should learn to eat as normally as possible after a fast.

Model of Luqaimat day
"Loqaimat diet system

Sample menu for 1-2 pounds of weight loss per week.

EXAMPL I:

2 Cup of water

3 Vanilla cinnamon + ½ cup of tea (1 teaspoon of sugar)

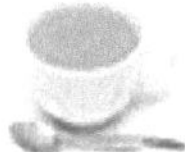

2 Cup of water, 3 Almonds or 5 peanuts

1 apple

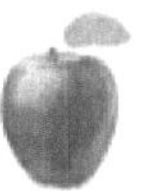

2 Cup of water, 3 Almonds or 5 peanuts

20 g chocolate

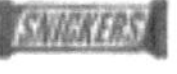

2 Cup of water, 3 Almonds or 5 peanuts

1.5 cup food + 1.5 cup of salad + 20g of ice cream

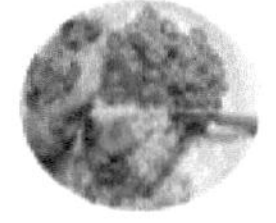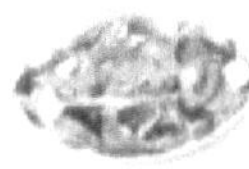

2 Cup of water, 3 Almonds or 5 peanuts

1 apple

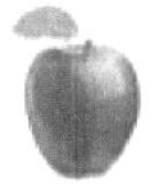

2 Cup of water, 3 Almonds or 5 peanuts

6 ounce container Greek yogurt + 10 blueberries + ¼ cup granola

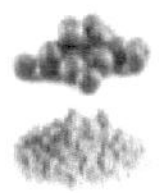

EXAMPL II:

2 Cup of water

1 Toast + Egg + ½ cup of Tea

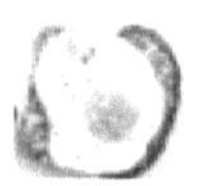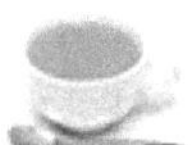

2 Cup of water, 3 Almonds or 5 peanuts

Banana

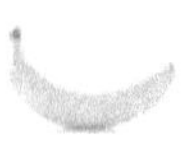

2 Cup of water, 3 Almonds or 5 peanuts

Hand sized lasagnas+ 1 cup of salad + ½ cup lemon juice.

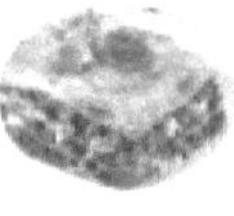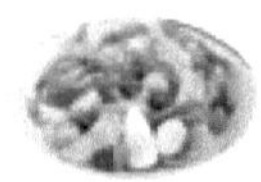

2 Cup of water, 3 Almonds or 5 peanuts

5 biscuits + cup of Green tea

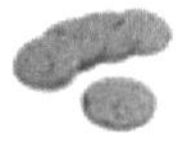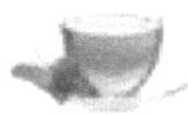

2 Cup of water, 3 Almonds or 5 peanuts

Banana

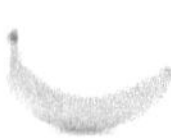

2 Cup of water, 3 Almonds or 5 peanuts

1 cup of yogurt

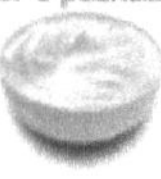

Start the diet of today

All you are required for a full month is to get rid of only 4lb and you will notice that despite the small amount of descent that your clothes began to expand on you.

This proves that the "science of Luqaimat" is different from the rest of the diet because it does not cause tension does not increase hormone cortisol, which causes increase of water and salts in the body and therefore the loss of 15-17lb takes you to two dimensions smaller.